Dedication

To my beautiful wife.

Thank you for Your patience

Table Of Contents

Chapter 1: Erectile dysfunction -What and Why?

We all are well aware and willing to discuss our health problems so that we remain in good physical form. Unfortunately, when it comes to our sexual performance / health we hardly tend to open up about the dysfunctions and irregularities. Nevertheless they hamper our sexual life to such extend which may be irreparable. It's well known that people suffering from such disorders develop an inferiority complex which often becomes the root cause of other *psychological and mental problems.*

Breaking the conventional idea, I wish to reach and convey to my readers that there should be no shying away from this issue. WE should treat this problem no different than the other diseases like diabetes, typhoid etc. The longer we hesitate in curing this problem, the stronger it becomes. People with this disease remain unknown, just because people **don't accept** the fact that they have sexual disorder. Please forget about your ego for a moment and start doing something about this. Buying this book is the first step.

Fortunately, Erectile Dysfunction is not just treatable, but also curable. Although, in order to get rid of it completely you have to address the underlying cause of the problem first. People don't like to admit it, but the main cause of Erectile Dysfunction is because of the lifestyle you've chosen. You won't be able to cure this problem, if you're not ready to make changes in your life.

Many people think that these disorders pass on from one generation to another or they symbolize lack of libido. These thoughts are nothing more than crap that keeps them away from coming out from the problem. They don't even believe that there's a cure. Thankfully, they're mistaken.

There are a lot of cases reported and yet the number awaits to triple fold if the unreported ones are also considered. Another thing to keep settle with is nothing is without a cause, if it happened to you it has a reason. So let's have a swift look on the possible causes that paves way to this highly uninvited circumstance.

Now it has been proven that male sexual excitements are a compiled process involving several factors like brain, hormones, emotions, nerves, muscles and blood vessels. When so many aspects influence the sexual arousal in men then they can obviously be hindered by any. But the most foreseen among them is stress or bad mental health as per reports is believed. Stress not only causes erectile dysfunction but at times worsen it to a highly dangerous level.

Very often psychological and physical issues have a combined result in form of sexual dysfunction. For example, if someone has been suffering from any physical pain that slows down sexual response may develop a kind of mental pressure blended with anxiety to hold an erection. In my opinion, anxiety is the main evil-doer of sexual dysfunction. There are other psychological problems spoiling the condition at its worst. It actually draws you to a *never-ending* cycle, when a male fails to perform sexually the atmosphere in the relationship gets soured at some point which puts you in a state of depression.

There are few listed diseases which are more than often responsible for this male sexual disorder. They are low testosterone, clogged blood vessels, diabetes, high cholesterols, obesity, heart disease, multiple sclerosis and Parkinson's disease. The other could be alcoholism, smoking, drug addiction, and tobacco. Having a healthy body really matters. Certain medications like treatment of prostate cancer and surgeries of pelvic areas or spinal cord are also the causes behind ED. There's one factor working on our favor - when we know the cause, curing it will not be a problem. I'll talk about that more in-depth in Chapter 4.

Losing the ability to obtain an erection is the biggest fear in men's life. Thank You for taking the first step towards improving your sexual life and therefore – improving your life in general.

Chapter 2: Recognize the problem.

Treatment of any disease depends upon two factors but first thing is recognizing the problem. Now when we know there could be more than one reason behind ED it's naturally expected that symptoms should vary depending upon the cause. So the problem is said to have abilities to manifest it in many ways. **There's a reason why you clicked on this book.**

Even if you don't have ED or if You don't want to admit it – you'll find the advices in this book very beneficial to your sexual health.

There nothing to lose, but everything to gain.

If *it* happens more or less transient or momentarily, there is nothing to worry about. Nearly all men face this at some point of their lives, but it is not serious and certainly you should not take much stress about it. Similarly is the dysfunction shows a gradual development and then seems to persist, you need to face it. In these conditions it is normally seen that physical reason are behind it and is called chronic impotence.

An erection problem when get associated with pain then it's something more serious, the diseased is called Peyronie's disease. The erectile dysfunction can be symptoms of other. When your mind indicates that there is any of the listed symptoms, don't waste time just run to the doctor. It is for your good and in long run could even prove vital in order to save your relationship.

"The first step in solving a problem is to recognize that it does exist."

- Zig Ziglar

Chapter 3: Why ED is Dangerous

More or less, each and every disorder has its own side effects with fewer exceptions. But the astonishing fact remains that even their treatments have some kind of effects that are not required on our body. ED is a serious sexual health issue so it certainly won't be life threatening or pose other physical problems .On the other hand it affects adversely on our mental status. It leads us to low self-esteem and depression due to the soured relationship when a person fails to perform while intercourse. And we all know that having low self-esteem and being in depressive state will cause other problems, that's why it's extremely important to deal with it.

Look its treatments have more complicated health problems on one's body at physical level than the disease itself. For example Viagra is drug used in its medication contains phosphodiesterase inhibitors. First and foremost warning, PDE should not be used by men who take medicine containing nitrates which is used to treat angina. Blood thinning medicine users, enlarged prostate and high BP patients should also keep caution rather take extra care with ED medicines. These issues should be discussed with your physician before starting treatment for erectile dysfunction. One more thing to remember, when PDE and these drugs interact they automatically pave way for physical agonies like head ache, nasal congestion, upset stomach plus hearing and vision problems.

A history of heart disease, uncontrolled diabetes, past or recent strokes and extremely low or very high BP patients are also advised to discuss the side effects of such treatments before starting it with their doctors in length. It is very important for complete well-being of your own body. After all we don't want cure a disease and get two more in return.

Your body is Your temple. Take a good care of it.

Chapter 4: Causes of Erectile Dysfunction

As I already mentioned in first Chapter, there are many causes of Erectile Dysfunction. Most of us are embarrassed to visit a doctor and talk about of disorder, we hope for a simple and instant cure in for of pill. Oftentimes, doctor will ask on a complete diagnosis to ensure that there are no serious health problems. ED doesn't come alone. It happens for a reason – there's something wrong with your physical or mental health.

The way we chose to lead our lives have direct effects on our health and body. They are kind of directive guidelines to what our body will be going through. A healthy lifestyle undoubtedly will positively impact on our body. This particular theory goes round the similar way so it's but natural that unhealthy lifestyle habits are going to bring something or other unwanted situation related to our overall well-being. It has been discovered that erectile dysfunction is caused or worsened in many men due to their wrong lifestyle choices. In my practice, undoing them could help a lot in the whole process of recovery.

There are main lifestyle factors and health conditions that are causing your dysfunction.

Obesity

You'll notice that adding a few more extra pounds will not only change your physique, but also change your state of mind. Being obese makes you sick, sad and depressed. Having a high body-fat percentage will cause Erectile Dysfunction. Your body will start to slow the production of testosterone. But *increase* production of estrogen, female sex hormone. You'll find it difficult to maintain an erection. There's a rumors that fat men last longer, but I totally disagree with that.

Diabetes

Can be caused by obesity and will negatively affect your whole body. It will elevate your sugar levels, men with diabetes have damaged nerves and different blood vessel problems, this means having erection problems is inevitable. Men with diabetes don't have problems with libido, unfortunately they're usually not hard enough for penetration or are not able to get an erection.

Heart Disease

A bad diet and lifestyle often leads to the hardening of your arteries as plaques form around blood vessel and it causes blood vessels to narrow, making it difficult for blood to pass through them. Usually, smaller blood vessels get affected first – the blood vessels leading to the penis. This is the reason why doctors very often see ED as an early sign of plaque appearance in the blood vessels. If you do not treat this problem, it might as well be *fatal.*

Pornography

I've decided to put this very high on the risk, because there's too much men who still watch pornography while being in the relationships. It not only drains your energy, affects your mentally and also **lowers your libido.** I've also suffered because of the pornography and I got problems getting excited by real sexual encounters. *I challenge you* do stop watching pornography for a month, you'll even see the difference in your sex-life within the first two weeks.

Smoking

Here's another reason to quit smoking, just by saying "no" to the cigarette will helps you to achieve firmer, harder, thicker and longer erections. The problems here is – smoking damages your blood vessels and interferes with blood flow. However, you might not realize how big of an impact cigarette has on your body. Thankfully, smoking does not cause extensive damage to your body. That does not apply if you've been smoking for the past few years, having a cigarette few times per month is totally okay.

Your penis and Your body will be grateful, when You quit inhaling the cigarette.

Alcoholism

Another common cause of Erectile Dysfunction, it could cause temporal problems, but can eventually lead to a long-term condition. And again, alcohol reduces blood flow not only to the brain, but to your penis as well. Men who drink alcohol tend to have weaker orgasm, lack of sexual desire and premature ejaculation. My advice on alcohol – drink only the **best quality** alcohol only and in moderation. A day after drinking you should cleanse your body, by drinking *at least* 4 liter of water.

Processed or low quality Foods

The American diet is filled with trans*fats, different preservatives, GMO foods and contain a lot of sugars. That's why we have young guys in their early 20's with Erectile Dysfunction. It's all over the internet, trans*fats are cause of different disorders, such as ED and obesity. Your body is unhealthy and weak on the inside. Your body is too busy removing all the junk, that's why procreative ability has to suffer.

Medications

There are many medications that could cause Erectile Dysfunction. For example Antidepressants (Prozac, for example), many different Cholesterol Lowering Drugs, Heartburn Medications. You should do your own research on this. Experts say that many different medications affect your hormones and neurotransmitters. Stick *to natural remedies* if you can.

Natural Cures for Erectile Dysfunction

The best part of this book. Thankfully, Erectile Dysfunction is curable and reversible. You're probably suffering this conditions because of health and lifestyle. In my opinion, your penis shows what's happening in the rest of the body. It shows the lack of balance between mind and body. When you get your health and life in balance, things will go smooth again. The sad news is, you'll have to make changes to your lifestyle.

Healthy Eating

Unfortunately, there's no such thing as a "magic food" that grants you strong and instant erections if you consume it in large quantity. In my experience, changing quality of your food at least for one week, will make you feel totally different. Keep your food consumption balance and emphasize on healthy, organic food items, while avoiding processed and low quality foods.

What should you eat?

Fruits – all fruits will be great for your body, but you'd want to choose ones high in vitamin C. Studies show, that regular consumption of vitamin C will drastically improve your sperm quality.

Green veggies – including lettuce, cabbage, spinach and more. Spinach contains large quantities of magnesium which will help with the dilation of blood vessels. Spinach are also rich in folate – substance that is linked to the prevention of plaque buildup in your blood vessels. Basically, they help with blood circulations, meaning, you'll have harder erections. I always eat 50g-100g of spinach a day. Add then to your salad!

Eggs – high in protein and contain many vitamins, eggs can help with weight loss. They balance hormones in your body and can boost the level of libido, regardless if you're male or female. My father in law drinks 5 **quail eggs** everyday (they do not contain salmonella, so you can use them raw) and always says that only because of this food he can have "erection like 20 year old" he's at his late 50. As from my experience, these eggs drastically increase my libido. They are high in cholesterol, which will help with testosterone production. I strongly suggest you do use 5 quail eggs everyday for a least a month, you'll definitely feel the difference.

Fish – fatty fish is good for you, not only because it has omega-3 fatty acids, but also because of the high contents of L-arginine – compound that boosts hormone production. In addition, you should supplement with high quality fish oil.

Dark Chocolate – There's a recent study found that flavonoids in dark chocolate can improve circulation. That could be good for erection problems that are due to poor circulation. Flavonoids are naturally- occurring antioxidants that protect plants from toxins and help repair cell damage. Studies show that flavonoids and other antioxidants have similar effects on people. They may help lower blood pressure and decrease cholesterol, both of which are factors that contribute to erectile dysfunction. The sad thing is, most chocolate in the market is filled with *many different preservatives.*

Other foods – **Red meat**, grass fed. Too much red meat could be bad for you. **Nuts**, peanuts are great source of healthy fats. A recent study found that men with erectile dysfunction who ate pistachio nuts every day for three weeks experienced significant improvement in sexual issues, including ED, sexual desire, and overall sexual satisfaction. **Berries,** fresh berries are one of the most *powerful disease-fighting* foods available, filled with many natural antioxidants.

Weight Lifting and Weight Loss

As a certified personal-trainer I've different opinion, unlike the most authors who write about this. They are not giving the best quality advice and sometimes their advice does more harm than good. Please understand, everything written is this book is very important, one change to your lifestyle **won't fix your condition.** But the weight-lifting and exercising definitely is the most impactful. After this book I'll be releasing more in-depth guide about exercising.

The effects of exercise on people with ED are awesome. For people who are obese / overweight, exercising not only will burn few pounds, but also decrease the chance of having heart disease and diabetes – also linked to Erectile Dysfunction.

If you're already in your ideal weight and have a healthy body-fat percentage, it's still a good idea to do different exercises, just to maintain your physique or boost your self-esteem. When you're confident about your looks, you'll have a fewer inhibitions in bed, that will result in more satisfying sex and intimacy with your partner. Exercising will improve your whole physique and treat any other health problem that you might have. Exercising will boost oxygen in the body, improve circulation of the blood and increase production of nitric oxide within your body. The reason why you get strong erections while being on Viagra is because of the nitric oxide. There's no need to use *blue pill,* you can get the same effect naturally.

It's well known, that testosterone, a male sex hormone, has a huge impact on a man's reproductive and sexual function. The best way to boost your T-levels naturally is to do weight-lifting. Lower the number of reps and increase the weight. If you've been doing body-building type routines all the time, heavy weight-lifting will also break plateau effect and you'll get more results.

Stick to the compound exercises that work large muscle groups, for example, squats, deadlifts. Yes, I known they're painful, but the reward is huge. You should ideally be using 80-95% of your 1RM (one rep max). Your goal should be 5-8 reps for 2-5 sets. Aim for 2-3 weight-lifting workouts per week, supplemented with 1-2 days of cardio. Studies have shown that **HIIT training,** bicycling, boxing, running can increase production of hormones and improve your mental health. Although, if you're a beginner, I strongly recommend you to hire a personal-trainer. There are a lot of young guys who would work with you for a cheap price, just to gain experience. Forget about your ego.

Quit Smoking

First and foremost thing, quit smoking! If you have trouble quitting try some professional help. Nicotine replacement like gum and lozenges would help you to get rid of the ill habit. This step is quite recommendable for complete goodness of your health and immunity. Let's be honest here, quitting smoking is not an easy job, but it's well-known about how much cigarette affects your body and sexual health. *Is it really worth it?*

This book is not about smoking, but I'll give you a template on how you should approach it. Before we start, I would like to guess why most people are smoking.

Process. You probably love the process of it. Putting the cigarette in your mouth, lighting in up and feeling *instant gratification.* I'll ask again, *is it really worth it?* The reward of not smoking is too high. You're using **external and <u>unnatural</u>** methods to feel relaxed, and what do you expect? You get **unnatural** response from your body, in a form of ED. Your body punishes you, because you harm it with your actions. If you love the process that much, there are a lot of techniques that you can use to feel relaxed. I could write a book about it, do your own research on this. Alternatively, you could use E-cigarette without preservatives and nicotine. I haven't used this personally, but my friends had a very good success with it.

People around You. Probably your co-worker, family members and friends are also smoking, and you go "with the flow" and have a smoke with them, just to feel closer to them. And when you say that you're quitting the cigarette they laugh at you or look at you in disbelief. They will try to affect you and your decision of quitting the nicotine. That's because, they want to **drag you down to their level.** They don't want you to surpass them, because it will show the weakness it themselves. Let's the honest, if you quit smoking that already indicates that you have *more* self-discipline and a stronger will-power than other smokers you know. Do your own conclusions. Period.

• Decide on a day you quit smoking.

• A week or two weeks before that day lower your consumption of nicotine.

• Fight the craving.

• Reward yourself for EACH day of resisting the temptation. Remember the quote, *What gets rewarded, gets repeated.*

• A healthy body already is a reward. A reward that money can't buy. But we all live in the material world, buy yourself a snack or go to the movies. It's up to you.

• Decide on a **punishment.** If you failed, you deserve to be punished. Decide on your own.

• Have an accountability partner. There's nothing wrong to ask for help. Just find a person who truly cares about you and your health. Your accountability can't be a smoker for obvious reasons.

• Have a smoke once in a while. I usually smoke cigar once per month just to relax myself even more. This way, I'm **NOT** being used by a substance, but using it myself. I'm *in control*, but smokers – are not, that's why they can't quit smoking. Period.

What Should You NOT Do

Processed and Fried Food Choices

This also means quitting fast-food, this includes hotdogs, sausages, bacon, burgers or anything else unhealthy. You'll find that these foods contain a very high amount of salt, sugar, preservatives and *low quality* carbohydrates. Yes, processed food is *much* cheaper than organic and healthy food, it's made on purpose. You should ask yourself is your health and well-being more important than a piece of paper. **Note:** I **strongly** suggest you to stop using vegetable oils, I personally use coconut oil or best quality olive oil. There are many different health benefits, just by consuming one teaspoon of coconut oil before breakfast will make the big difference.

Alcohol Consumption

Let's be honest, alcohol is a depressant, it can decrease your sexual desire, make you depressed, make it hard to achieve erection. The totally different effect can be achieved if it's used *in moderation.* Moderation is the key, the same things is with smoking – **you have to be in control.** I'll even further, you suffer them Erectile Dysfunction, because **YOU'RE NOT IN CONTROL.** If you are not able to control your life, then how do you expect to control **your penis?** Don't get offended. You'll not read anything like this in other books – other authors don't want to help you.

Sleep

Sleep deprivation is a torture for your body, it pushes person's psychological and mental well-being the edge. Being tired will not make you want to have sex, you might be ready mentally, but your body will be drained, you'll have a *hard* time attaining an erection. **Note:** if you're experimenting with polyphasic sleep schedule, make sure that you're healthy enough. Meaning, your nutrition, lifestyle have to be balanced.

Here's some techniques you can use to have a better sleep:

• Avoid computers, TV, mobile phone an hour before sleep.

• Don't drink coffee 4 hours before bed.

• Listen to audiobook or read a book in your bed.

• Make sure your room is *completely dark,* only exception is candle light.

• Don't eat too much before bed.

• Based on my experience, protein and fats will help you to fall asleep faster. I usually start and end my day with fat/protein meals. *Why do you need carbs in your sleep?*

Herbs and Supplements

There are many herbs and supplements that will help you with your condition. Not only good for your sexual health, but also for your overall health. I suggest to use them in the purest form, because you might never know how other preservatives could affect you. If a label is too fancy – don't buy it. Don't buy overpriced supplements – there really isn't much of a difference. You could save even more money by buying directly from the manufacturer. Without the further due, let's continue.

L - Arginine

Very useful amino acid, especially if you're going to the gym. It helps with blood circulatory problems, regulates blood pressure and prevents heart disease. Your body needs a little help, because it doesn't pump enough blood into your penis, that's why you experience no erection. This amino acid is in foods such as **pumpkin seeds, peanuts, walnuts.** Also **Garlic** help with blood flow. I eat a lot of garlic with my foods, that's why I don't use salt, ketchup or anything else.

Horny Goat Weed

This is extremely legit herb. This substance is always used in Testosterone boosters and in other "Man's Health" related supplements. Horny goat weed will give you similar effect that

Viagra does. Just don't overuse it. It's very cheap and available everywhere. From my experience – use it 5 hours before sex.

Hawthorn Berry and Cayenne

Both will help you with blood circulation and will make you **extra hard.** I still sometimes buy these, just to give my woman even more pleasure. Very easy to buy online and is available in capsules. **Do not overuse.**

Disclaimer: I'm not a doctor. Consult with the doctor about how these substances could affect your health. What works for me, might not work for you.

Conclusion

At the end I'll say you that Erectile Dysfunction is easy to stay away from. All you need is awareness and understanding that it is just another disease which you can deal with easily. Beside it is also quite rare to get entangled in the web of ED once you have been out of the situation. Your doctor will make sure from his side but do your bit too for a healthy lifestyle. Although, it's up to you to conquer this challenge. If I could do that, so can **YOU! I have total faith in You!**

Good luck my friends!

Finally, if you enjoyed this book, then I'd like to ask you for a favor, would you be kind enough to leave a review for this book on Amazon? It'd be greatly appreciated! Also feel free to check out my other books.

Thank You !

Huge Thank You and Words of Gratitude!

First and foremost, Thank You for downloading this book. At the end of the day I'm **extremely** grateful for **every** download and **every** purchase. It really makes me smile and motivates me. I wish that every person would put their best forward for the human race. I wish you unlimited mental strength and discipline to achieve your goals and dreams. **Together** we can make the difference.

Copyright

clarifying purposes only and are owned by the owners themselves, not affiliated with this document.